Berthold Koletzko, Kathrin Krohn, Olivier Goulet, Raanan Shamir

Paediatric Parenteral Nutrition

A Practical Reference Guide

13 tables, 2008

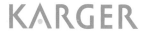
KARGER

Basel · Freiburg · Paris · London · New York · Bangalore
Bangkok · Shanghai · Singapore · Tokyo · Sydney

Berthold Koletzko, MD, Professor
of Paediatrics
Division of Metabolic Diseases and
Nutritional Medicine
Dr. von Hauner Children's Hospital
Ludwig Maximilian University
DE–80337 Munich (Germany)
office.koletzko@med.uni-muenchen.de

Olivier Goulet, MD, Professor
of Paediatrics
Department of Pediatric Gastroenterology,
Hepatology and Nutrition
Center for Rare Digestive Diseases
Hôpital Necker – Enfants Malades
University of Paris
FR–75015 Paris (France)

Kathrin Krohn, MD
Division of Metabolic Diseases and
Nutritional Medicine
Dr. von Hauner Children's Hospital
Ludwig Maximilian University
DE–80337 Munich (Germany)

Raanan Shamir, MD
Institute of Gastroenterology, Nutrition
and Liver Diseases
Schneider Children's Medical Center
Tel Aviv University
Tel Aviv 49202 (Israel)
raanans@clalit.org.il

Sponsored by an unrestricted educational grant from Baxter.
Baxter was not involved in the development or review of the content of
the book.

Library of Congress Cataloging-in-Publication Data

Paediatric parenteral nutrition : a practical reference guide / Berthold
Koletzko ... [et al.].
    p. ; cm.
  Includes bibliographical references.
  ISBN 978-3-8055-8606-1 (soft cover : alk. paper)
  1. Parenteral feeding of children--Handbooks, manuals, etc. I. Koletzko,
B. (Berthold)
  [DNLM: 1. Parenteral Nutrition--Handbooks. 2. Child. 3. Infant. WB 39
P126 2008]
  RJ53.P37P33 2008
  618.92--dc22
                        2008021108

Drug Dosage. The authors and the publisher have exerted every effort to ensure that drug selection and
dosage set forth in this text are in accord with current recommendations and practice at the time of publication. However, in view of ongoing research, changes in government regulations, and the constant flow
of information relating to drug therapy and drug reactions, the reader is urged to check the package insert
for each drug for any change in indications and dosage and for added warnings and precautions. This is
particularly important when the recommended agent is a new and/or infrequently employed drug.

© Copyright 2008 by S. Karger AG, P.O. Box, CH–4009 Basel (Switzerland)
www.karger.com
Printed in Switzerland on acid-free paper by Reinhardt Druck, Basel
ISBN 978–3–8055–8606–1

Paediatric Parenteral Nutrition

A Practical Reference Guide

This book is due for return on or before the last date shown below.

Contents

Introduction

This compact reference booklet on parenteral nutrition (PN) in children is based on the Guidelines for Paediatric Parenteral Nutrition that have been developed jointly by the European Society for Paediatric Gastroenterology, Hepatology and Nutrition (www.espghan.org) and the European Society for Clinical Nutrition and Metabolism (www.espen.org) in collaboration with the European Society for Paediatric Research (www.espr.org) [1]. These guidelines were developed based on systematic literature reviews and a formal consensus process by a multidisciplinary working party of professionals, who are all actively involved in the management of children treated with PN (cf. list of contributors). As a result of the scarcity of good quality clinical trials in children, many of the recommendations are extrapolated from adult studies and are based on expert opinion. A detailed analysis of the available data was performed and for each statement the level of evidence (table 1) and grade of recommendation (table 2) was assessed.

The *Guidelines* are intended to serve as an aid to clinical judgement, not to replace it. The ultimate decision about the clinical management of an individual patient should always depend on the clinical circumstances (and wishes) of the patient, and on the clinical judgement of the healthcare team.

This handbook presents a very condensed version of the *Guidelines for Paediatric Parenteral Nutrition.* More detailed information can be found in the original publication [1] which is available at www.espghan.org

Indications for PN

PN is required if nutritional needs cannot be met by oral or enteral feeding. The initiation of PN will depend both on individual circumstances and the age and size of the infant or child. In the small preterm infant starvation for just one day may be detrimental, and where it is clear that enteral feeds will not be tolerated soon, PN must be instituted shortly after birth. However in older children and in adolescents longer periods of inadequate nutrition of up to about 7 days may be tolerated, depending on age, nutritional status, and the disease, surgical or medical intervention.

Table 1. Grading of levels of evidence (LOE) according to the Scottish Intercollegiate Guideline Network 2000

1++	High-quality meta-analyses, systematic reviews of randomised controlled trials (RCTs), or RCTs with a very low risk of bias
1+	Well-conducted meta-analyses, systematic reviews of RCTs, or RCTs with a low risk of bias
1−	Meta-analyses, systematic reviews of RCTs, or RCTs with a high risk of bias
2++	High-quality systematic reviews of case-control or cohort studies High-quality case-control or cohort studies with a very low risk of confounding, bias, or chance and a high probability that the relationship is causal
2+	Well-conducted case-control or cohort studies with a low risk of confounding, bias, or chance and a moderate probability that the relationship is causal
2−	Case-control or cohort studies with a high risk of confounding, bias, or chance and a significant risk that the relationship is not causal
3	Non-analytic studies, e.g. case reports, case series Evidence from non-analytic studies, e.g. case reports, case series
4	Evidence from expert opinion

Table 2. Grading of recommendations (GOR) according to the Scottish Intercollegiate Guideline Network 2000

A	Requires at least one meta-analysis, systematic review or RCT rated as 1++, and directly applicable to the target population; or a systematic review of RCTs, or a body of evidence consisting principally of studies rated as 1+, directly applicable to the target population and demonstrating overall consistency of results
B	Requires a body of evidence including studies rated as 2++, directly applicable to the target population, and demonstrating overall consistency of results; or extrapolated evidence from studies rated as 1++ or 1+
C	Requires a body of evidence including studies rated as 2+, directly applicable to the target population and demonstrating overall consistency of results; or extrapolated evidence from studies rated as 2++
D	Evidence level 3 or 4; or extrapolated evidence from studies rated as 2+

Co-Authors of the ESPGHAN/ESPEN Guidelines on Paediatric Parenteral Nutrition (in alphabetical order)

Carlo Agostoni, Milan, Italy
Patrick Ball, Auckland, New Zealand
Virgilio Carnielli, Ancona, Italy
Chris Chaloner, Manchester, UK
Jane Clayton, Manchester, UK
Virginie Colomb, Paris, France
Monique Dijsselhof, Amsterdam,
     The Netherlands
Christoph Fusch, Greifswald, Germany
Paolo Gandullia, Genoa, Italy
Orsolya Genzel-Boroviczeny
     Munich, Germany
Frédéric Gottrand, Lille, France
Olivier Goulet, Paris, France
Esther Granot, Jerusalem, Israel
James Gray, Birmingham, UK
Antonio Guerra, Porto, Portugal
Susan Hill, London, UK
Chris Holden, Birmingham, UK
Venetia Horn, London, UK
Joanne Hunt, Munich, Germany
Loveday Jago, Manchester, UK
Frank Jochum, Berlin, Germany
Sanja Kolacek, Zagreb, Croatia
Berthold Koletzko, Munich, Germany
Sibylle Koletzko, Munich, Germany
Kathrin Krohn, Munich, Germany

Janusz Ksiazyk, Warsaw, Poland
Alexandre Lapillonne, Paris, France
Päivi Luukkainen, Helsinki, Finland
Malgorzata Lyszkowska, Warsaw, Poland
Sarah MacDonald, London, UK
Julije Meštroviæ, Split, Croatia
Walter Mihatsch, Schwäbisch Hall,
     Germany
Peter Milla, London, UK
Francis Mimouni, Tel Aviv, Israel
Zrinjka Mišak, Zagreb, Croatia
Irena Mršic, Zagreb, Croatia
Liz Newby, Liverpool, UK
Frank Pohlandt, Ulm, Germany
Sue Protheroe, Birmingham, UK
John Puntis, Leeds, UK
Jacques Rigo, Liège, Belgium
Arieh Riskin, Haifa, Israel
Jane Roberts, Manchester, UK
Raanan Shamir, Haifa, Israel
Peter Szitanyi, Prague, Czech Republic
Adrian Thomas, Manchester, UK
Nachum Vaisman, Tel Aviv, Israel
Hans van Goudoever, Rotterdam,
     The Netherlands
Ayala Yaron, Tel Aviv, Israel

Energy

Energy supply should aim at covering the nutritional needs of the patient (basal metabolic rate, physical activity, growth and correction of pre-existing malnutrition) including the support of anabolic functions [2]. Excessive energy intake as well as underfeeding may lead to complications [3, 4]. Generally, energy needs are higher in enteral nutrition (EN) compared to PN. Theoretically, energy needs can be calculated based on non-protein calories as protein needs are calculated only for maintenance and tissue deposit and not as an energy source. For practical reasons and uniformity, most statements in this chapter refer to total energy supply including proteins.

Premature Infants

Early nutrition support is advocated in extremely low birth weight (ELBW) and very low birth weight (VLBW) infants because of limited nutritional stores [5]. Energy intake affects nitrogen balance; minimal energy requirements are met with 50–60 kcal/kg per day, but 100–120 kcal/kg per day facilitate maximal protein accretion and growth [6]. A neonate receiving PN needs fewer calories (90–100 kcal/kg per day) than an enterally fed infant because there is no energy lost in the stools and there is less thermogenesis [7].

Post-Operative Needs

Most of the studies indicate that major operations such as abdominal surgery are not accompanied by increased energy expenditure [8]. It is not necessary to increase the energy intake of infants who have an uncomplicated operation [7].

— Energy intake should be adapted in patients with disease states that increase resting energy expenditure, such as pulmonary (e.g. cystic fibrosis) and cardiac (e.g. some congenital heart diseases) disorders. **GOR B**

— Energy intake should not be increased after uncomplicated surgery. **GOR B**

— Total parenteral energy needs (including protein) of stable patients may be roughly estimated using the following table. **GOR D**

Age, years	kcal/kg body weight per day
Preterm	110–120
0–1	90–100
1–7	75–90
7–12	60–75
12–18	30–60

Amino Acids

Amino acid requirements are lower in parenterally fed infants and children than in enterally fed infants because the supply bypasses the intestine. There is a wide variation in the intestinal uptake and utilisation of specific amino acids that changes with age. Recommended intakes for different age groups are presented here. Details on administration and metabolism of specific amino acids are provided in the *Guidelines* [1].

Recommendations

— Recommended parenteral amino acid supply per day. **GOR D**

Age		Comment
Preterms	1.5–4 g/kg	Amino acid supply should start on the first postnatal day. **GOR B** For tissue growth more than 1.5 g/kg per day are required.
Term neonates	1.5–3 g/kg	
Infants to 2nd year	1–2.5 g/kg	
3rd to 18th year	1–2 g/kg	For critically ill patients the advisable amino acid intake may be higher (up to 3 g/kg per day). **GOR D**

Lipid Emulsions

Fat oxidation depends on the total energy intake and expenditure, the total intake of carbohydrates and triglycerides and the carbohydrate/fat ratio administered [9, 10] (LOE 1). As carbohydrate intake increases, fat oxidation is reduced and lipid storage enhanced.

Recommendations

— Lipid emulsions are an integral part of paediatric PN providing a high energy supply without carbohydrate overload and they supply essential fatty acids. **GOR D**

— Lipid intake should usually provide **25–40% of non-protein calories** in fully parenterally fed patients. **GOR D**

— Glucose intakes above 18 g/kg per day, which tend to induce net lipogenesis in infants, should usually be avoided in infants. **GOR B**

Fat Intake

Omission of lipid emulsions from total PN may lead to biochemical evidence of essential fatty acid deficiency within a few days in preterm infants [11–13].

The upper limit of lipid administration is difficult to determine. In preterm infants a lipid supply of 3 g/kg per day as continuous infusion was tolerated well, based on measurement of serum triglycerides, cholesterol and molar ratios of free fatty acids/albumin [14–16]. However, preterm infants weighing less than 1,000 g deserve special attention because their tolerance to intravenous lipids may be limited [17] (LOE 2–3).

In term infants fat oxidation reaches a maximum at 4 g/kg per day, given that the maximum glucose intake does not exceed maximal oxidative glucose disposal of about 18 g/kg per day [9, 10]. However, particularly in premature and VLBW infants, a lipid supply exceeding fat oxidation may be desirable to achieve fat deposition.

- In order to prevent essential fatty acid deficiency a **minimum linoleic acid intake** of **0.25 g/kg per day** should be given to **preterm infants** and **0.1 g/kg per day to term infants and older children (GOR D)**. When prescribing lipid emulsions the different linoleic acid content of the available lipid emulsions needs to be taken into account.
- Parenteral lipid intake should usually be limited to a **maximum of 3–4 g/kg per day** (0.13–0.17 g/kg per hour) in **infants (GOR B)** and **2–3 g/kg per day** (0.08–0.13 g/kg per hour) in **older children. GOR D**

Application

In preterm infants tolerance of lipid emulsions is improved by continuous infusion over 24 h versus an intermittent regime with lipid-free intervals [14, 16, 18]. Although there are no comparable studies in older children, continuous infusion of lipid emulsions along with the other PN components is recommended.

There is no evidence that gradual increments in the infusion rate of lipids improve fat tolerance [18]. An incremental increase in lipid infusion of 0.5–1 g/kg per day may help to identify fat intolerance (hypertriglyceridaemia) earlier at lower fat intake.

Clearance of lipid emulsions from the blood depends on the activity of lipoprotein lipase. Post-heparin lipoprotein lipase activity can be increased by relatively high doses of heparin [19, 20]. However, heparin does not improve utilisation of intravenous lipids [20–22].

- Dosage of lipid emulsions should not exceed the capacity for lipid clearance and should be adapted if marked hyperlipidaemia occurs. **GOR B**
- In infants, newborns and premature babies lipid emulsions should usually be administered continuously over about 24 h **(GOR B)**. If cyclic PN is used, for example in home PN, lipid emulsions should be given over the same duration as the other PN components. **GOR D**
- Heparin does not improve utilisation of intravenous lipids and should not be added to lipid infusion on a routine basis unless indicated for other reasons. **GOR B**

Monitoring

It is unclear at what serum triglyceride levels adverse effects may occur [23]. In premature and term infants triglyceride levels of 250 mg/dl during lipid infusion seem to be acceptable (LOE 4). For older children, a limit of 300–400 mg/dl may be acceptable based on the fact that lipoprotein lipase is saturated at around 400 mg/dl [24] (LOE 4).

Recommendations

— Triglyceride levels in serum or plasma should be monitored in patients receiving lipid emulsions, particularly in cases with a marked risk for hyperlipidaemia (e.g. patients with high lipid dosage, sepsis, catabolism, ELBW infants). **GOR D**

— Reduction in the dosage of lipid emulsions should be considered if serum or plasma triglyceride concentrations during infusion exceed **250 mg/dl in infants** or **400 mg/dl in older children. GOR D**

Available Lipid Emulsions

Statement and Recommendations

— The use of commercial lipid emulsions based on LCT (soybean oil or olive oil/soybean oil), or physical mixtures of MCT and LCT can be considered generally safe in infants and children. **LOE 1**

— There is currently no evidence (based on clinical outcome data) supporting the advantage of any of the lipid emulsions that are currently available [25]. **GOR D**

— Lipid emulsions used should not contain a higher phospholipid/triglyceride ratio than standard 20% lipid solutions in order to decrease the risk of hyperlipidaemia [26–28]. **GOR B**

Premature and Newborn Infants

Intravenous lipids may be well tolerated from the first day of life onwards [29]. However, early administration of lipid emulsions remains controversial because of the possibility of adverse effects on subsequent chronic lung disease (CLD) and mortality.

A meta-analysis designed to assess the effect of early (days 1–5) versus late (days 5–14) introduction of intravenous lipids reported no effect on the incidence of death or CLD at 28 days or at 36 weeks post-conception [30]. However, there are concerns about potential adverse effects of early administration of lipid emulsions in VLBW infants weighing less than 800 g [31].

The exposure of lipid solutions to phototherapy light may result in the formation of triglyceride hydroperoxides that may be harmful, especially to premature infants. Thus, lipid emulsions should always be protected from phototherapy light by special light-protected dark tubing [32] (LOE 2).

Statements and Recommendations

— In newborn infants who cannot receive sufficient enteral feeding, intravenous lipid emulsions should be started **no later than on the 3rd day** of life, but may be started on the **1st day** of life. **GOR B**

— Early administration of intravenous lipids in the first days of life does not increase the incidence of chronic lung disease or death in premature infants when compared to late administration of intravenous lipids **(LOE 1)**. However there are concerns about potential adverse effects of early administration of lipid emulsions in VLBW infants weighing less than 800 g. **LOE 2**

— Lipid emulsions have not been demonstrated to have a significant effect on hyperbilirubinaemia in populations of premature infants [33, 34] **(LOE 2)**. To limit the risk of increasing hyperbilirubinaemia lipid emulsions should be administered as continuous infusions [33]. It is unclear which level of bilirubin can be considered as safe in premature infants. In parenterally fed infants at risk of hyperbilirubinaemia, serum triglyceride and bilirubin levels should be monitored and the lipid infusion rate be adjusted if deemed necessary. **GOR D**

— Lipid emulsions should be protected by validated light-protected tubing during phototherapy to decrease the formation of hydroperoxides. **GOR B**

Carnitine

Currently PN solutions do not contain carnitine. Controversy exists as to the need to provide a source of carnitine to infants receiving total PN. A Cochrane-based meta-analysis showed no benefit of parenteral carnitine supplementation on lipid tolerance, ketogenesis or weight gain in neonates requiring PN [26] (LOE 1).

Statements and Recommendation

— Decreased levels of carnitine occur during prolonged PN without carnitine supplementation [35]. **LOE 1**

— There is no documented benefit of parenteral carnitine supplementation on lipid tolerance, ketogenesis or weight gain of neonates requiring PN. **LOE 1**

— Carnitine supplementation should be considered on an individual basis in patients receiving PN for more than 4 weeks. **GOR D**

Carbohydrates

Consequences of Overfeeding with Glucose

When glucose is administered in excess of the amount that can be directly oxidised for energy production and glycogen, the excess is directed to lipogenesis thus promoting fat deposition [5, 36]. This accounts, in part, for the increase in energy expenditure observed with high rates of glucose infusion [37]. Excessive glucose intake is thought to increase CO_2 production and minute ventilation [38–40]. Total energy delivery as well as amino acid intake also contributes to increased CO_2 production and minute ventilation [39, 40].

> **Statements**
>
> — Excessive glucose intake may induce hyperglycaemia. **LOE 1**
> — Excessive glucose intake causes increased lipogenesis and fat tissue deposition together with subsequent liver steatosis and enhanced production of VLDL triglycerides by the liver. **LOE 2–3**
> — Excessive glucose intake causes increased CO_2 production and minute ventilation. **LOE 3**
> — Excessive glucose intake causes impaired protein metabolism. **LOE 2–3**

Rate of Endogenous Glucose Production and Rate of Glucose Oxidation

The basal rate of glucose production varies from 8 mg/kg per min in preterm infants to 2 mg/kg per min in adults (or from 11.5 to 3 g/kg per day) [41–44]. The rate of glucose production is maximal during the postnatal period and decreases gradually with age. Gluconeogenesis provides a significant amount of glucose, and is responsible for about 31% of the rate of glucose appearance in healthy full-term newborns [41].

During high rates of glucose infusion, there is complete suppression of endogenous production of glucose accompanied by hyperinsulinism.

During PN glucose delivery should be kept constant without exceeding the maximum rate of glucose oxidation (RGO), which differs significantly among patients. Except for preterm infants, one could consider that maximal RGO is continuously decreasing from birth to adulthood. In appropriate for gestational age preterm infants, the RGO does not exceed 6–8 mg/kg per min (8.6–11.5 g/kg per day) after birth [45, 46] while in term surgical infants or infants on long-term PN, the maximal RGO is about 12 mg/kg per min (17.2 g/kg per day) [47, 48]. A study in critically burned children demonstrated the maximal RGO to be 5 mg/kg per min [49]. The clinical approach is to exercise restraint in the delivery of glucose in critically ill children.

Recommendations

- In preterm infants glucose intake should be started with 4–8 mg/kg per min (5.7–11.5 g/kg per day). **GOR C**
- Glucose administration to full-term neonates and children up to 2 years of age should not exceed 13 mg/kg per min (18.7 g/kg per day). **GOR C**
- In critically ill children glucose intake should be limited to 5 mg/kg per min (7.2 g/kg per day). **GOR D**
- Variations in glucose intake according to age and clinical situation (e.g. malnutrition, acute illness, drug administration) should be considered. **GOR D**
- Glucose intake should be adapted in case of simultaneous administration of drugs known to impair glucose metabolism such as steroids, somatostatin analogues, tacrolimus. **GOR C**
- Recommended glucose supply (g/kg body weight per day) **GOR D**

Weight	Day 1	Day 2	Day 3	Day 4
<3 kg	10	14	16	18
3–10 kg	8	12	14	16–18
10–15 kg	6	8	10	12–14
15–20 kg	4	6	8	10–12
20–30 kg	4	6	8	<12
>30 kg	3	5	8	<10

- These recommendations need to be adapted to the clinical situation (e.g. re-feeding syndrome in severe malnutrition), to oral and/or enteral energy intake and to the required weight gain for normal or catch-up growth. **GOR C**
- It is important, especially in infants, to accurately evaluate the carbohydrate load provided by concurrent infusion therapy. **GOR C**

cheal intubation and mechanical ventilation using warmed and humidified air significantly reduce insensible respiratory water [60] and the needs for fluids are reduced up to 20 ml/kg body weight per day.

> **Recommendation**
>
> — Phase II (stabilisation) when extracellular fluid compartment contraction is completed may vary in duration from about 5 to 15 days and is completed when birth weight is regained and the kidneys produce more concentrated urine. Expected weight gain is 10–20 g/kg body weight per day (table 4). **GOR D**

Table 4. Fluid and electrolyte supply during the intermediate phase

Birth weight	Fluid intake ml/kg body weight per day	Na+ intake mmol/kg body weight per day	K+ intake mmol/kg body weight per day	Cl- intake mmol/kg body weight per day
Term neonate	140–170	2.0–5.0	1.0–3.0	2.0–3.0
>1,500 g	140–160	3.0–5.0	1.0–3.0	3.0–5.0
<1,500 g	140–180	2.0–3.0 (5)	1.0–2.0	2.0–3.0

Phase III: Stable Growth

Stable growth is characterised by continuous weight gain with a positive net balance for water and sodium. Fluid requirement during phase III (table 5) is related to the expected weight gain.

> **Recommendation**
>
> — During phase III (established stable growth) the aim is to match physiological growth rates. Chloride supplementation follows sodium and potassium. Expected weight gain is 10–20 g/kg body weight per day (table 5). **GOR D**

Table 5. Fluid and electrolyte supply during the phase of stable growth

	Fluid intake ml/kg body weight per day	Na$^+$ intake mmol/kg body weight per day	K$^+$ intake mmol/kg body weight per day
Term neonate	140–160	2.0–3.0	1.5–3.0
Preterm neonate	140–160	3.0–5.0 (7.0)	2.0–5.0

Infants beyond the Neonatal Period and Children

Requirements on electrolytes for infants and children are based on empirical evidence [61] (GOR D) (tables 6 and 7). Daily maintenance fluid requirement is a function of total caloric expenditure at rest; for infants below 10 kg body weight it equals about 100 ml/kg body weight per day. Children with a body weight of 11–20 kg should receive 1,000 ml + 50 ml for each kg body weight above 10 kg, and children with a body weight above 20 kg should receive 1,500 ml + 20 ml for each kg above 20 kg [61] (GOR D).

Water requirements increase with fever, hyperventilation, hypermetabolism and gastrointestinal losses and decrease with, e.g., congestive heart failure.

Recommendation

Table 6. Electrolyte supply to infants beyond the neonatal period and children

Electrolyte	Infants	Children >1 year
Na$^+$, mmol/kg body weight per day	2.0–3.0	1.0–3.0
K$^+$, mmol/kg body weight per day	1.0–3.0	1.0–3.0

K$^+$ supplementation should usually start after onset of diuresis.

> — Parenterally fed infants and children should receive a daily iodine supply of 1 µg/kg per day. **GOR D**

Manganese

High Mn intake during PN is probably one of several factors contributing to the pathogenesis of PN-associated cholestasis or other hepatic dysfunction [76] (LOE 3); [73, 77] (LOE 2++); [78] (LOE 1). Mn should, therefore, be carefully administered, particularly in patients receiving long-term PN [73] (LOE 2++); [79] (LOE 3); [80] (LOE 2+). Studies using magnetic resonance images (MRIs) have reported high-intensity areas in basal ganglia, thalamus, brainstem and cerebellum due to Mn intoxication, with disappearance of symptoms and MRI abnormalities after withdrawal of Mn administration [81] (LOE 2+); [79, 82, 83] (LOE 3). Since central nervous system deposition of Mn can occur without symptoms, regular monitoring of Mn blood concentration should be carried out in children on long-term PN. A low-dose regimen of no more than 1.0 µg (0.018 µmol)/kg per day (maximum of 50 µg/day for children) is recommended [68, 73] (LOE 2++) together with regular examination of the nervous system [73].

Recommendation

> — In children receiving long-term PN, a low dose supply of Mn of no more than 1.0 µg (0.018 µmol)/kg per day (maximum of 50 µg/day for children) is recommended. **GOR D**

Molybdenum

Intravenous Mo supplements are recommended only with long-term PN.

Recommendations

> — An intravenous Mo supply of 1 µg/kg per day (0.01 µmol/kg per day) seems adequate and is recommended for LBW infants. **GOR D**
> — For infants and children an intravenous Mo supply of 0.25 µg/kg per day (up to a maximum of 5.0 µg/day) is recommended. **GOR D**

Selenium

It has been recommended that the plasma and red cell Se concentration and Se-dependent glutathione peroxidase (Se-GSHPx) are monitored in children receiving PN [84] (LOE 3).

A dose of 2–3 µg/kg per day has been recommended for LBW infants, although the optimal form and dose remain unclear [68, 85, 86] (LOE 2++). Premature infants (particularly the VLBW) might require twice the currently recommended Se intake of 2–3 µg/kg per day.

> **Recommendation**
>
> — An intravenous Se supply of 2–3 µg/kg per day is recommended for parenterally fed LBW infants. **GOR D**

Zinc

Premature infants need a higher Zn intake than term infants because of their rapid growth: 450–500 µg/kg per day to match the in utero accretion rate [87] (LOE 2+). Standard trace element preparations do not supply this amount, and additional Zn (Zn sulphate) may need to be added to PN fluid in the preterm infant, or those patients with high Zn losses e.g. from diarrhoea, stomal losses, severe skin disease [88] (LOE 2+) or following thermal injury [75] (LOE 2+). Zn is the only trace element that should be added to solutions of patients receiving short-term PN [68].

> **Recommendations**
>
> — Parenteral Zn supply is recommended in daily dosages of 450–500 µg/ kg per day for premature infants, 250 µg/kg per day for infants less than 3 months, 100 µg/kg per day for infants aged 3 months or older, and 50 µg/kg per day (up to a maximum of 5.0 mg/day) for children. **GOR D**
>
> — Excessive cutaneous or digestive losses of Zn require additional supplementation. **GOR D**

Vitamin K

Current multivitamin preparations contain high amounts of vitamin K which tend to supply 100 μg/kg (10 times higher than the recommended enteral intake), but adverse clinical effects have not been reported. A parenteral vitamin K supply of 80 μg/kg per day [115] in premature infants might be excessive if combined with an i.m. dosage of 1 mg on day 1, and lower supplies may suffice during the first weeks of life.

The suggested daily intake for children is 200 μg/day.

Statement and Recommendations

— Ranges of reasonable parenteral vitamin supply for infants and children are given in table 9. **GOR D**

— There are substantial losses of vitamin A when given with a water-soluble solution; therefore parenteral lipid-soluble vitamins should be given with the lipid emulsion whenever possible. **GOR D**

— For preterm infants, serum tocopherol levels should be between 1 and 2 mg/dl **(GOR A)**. To properly assess vitamin E status, the ratio between serum vitamin E and total serum lipids should be used.

— In exclusively parenterally fed infants a vitamin D supply of 30 IU/kg per day may be sufficient. **GOR D**

— A parenteral vitamin K supply of 80 μg/kg per day in premature infants might be excessive if combined with an i.m. dosage of 1 mg on day 1. **LOE 2**

Table 9. Recommended intakes for parenteral supply of lipid-soluble vitamins for infants and children [68, 112, 114, 115, 121–123]

	Infants, dose/kg body weight per day	Children, dose per day
Vitamin A, µg[a]	150–300	150
Vitamin D, µg	0.8 (32 IU)	10 (400 IU)
Vitamin E, mg	2.8–3.5	7
Vitamin K, µg	10 (recommended, but currently not possible)[b] if also given i.m. at birth	200

[a] 1 µg retinol equivalent = 1 µg all-trans retinol = 3.33 IU vitamin A.
[b] Current multivitamin preparations supply higher vitamin K amounts without apparent adverse clinical effects.

Water-Soluble Vitamins

Water-soluble vitamins must be administered on a regular basis as they are not stored in significant amounts, except for B_{12}. Excess is excreted by the kidneys and there is little toxicity. Term infants and children appear to adapt to large variations in vitamin intakes. By contrast, the finding of a marked elevation of some vitamins and low levels of others seen in infants below 1,500 g suggests that this group has less adaptive capacity to high- or low-dose intakes [116, 117].

Thiamine

Thiamine is excreted by the kidneys and toxicity is rarely detected. In parenterally fed infants and children a deficient thiamine supply may lead to severe lactic acidosis and even death within a period of only days to weeks [118]. The current parenteral recommendation for preterm infants (200–350 µg/kg per day) might be too low and dosages up to 500 µg/kg per day seem more appropriate [119], but further information is required.

— Where possible a central venous line should be dedicated for the administration of PN. **GOR B**

— If a CVC is used to administer PN, use a catheter with the minimal number of ports or lumens essential for the management of the patient. **GOR B**

— If a multi-lumen catheter is used to administer PN, designate one port exclusively for PN. Blood administration and central intravenous pressure monitoring from the designated line should be avoided. **GOR B** (from adult studies)

— If single lumen catheters are used, the risk of complications increases with blood sampling from the catheter. **GOR B** (from adult studies). However, to improve the quality of life of patients on long-term or home PN, blood sampling could be done from single-lumen catheters, provided that the procedure is aseptic. **LOE 4**

Catheter Heparinisation

The current attitude towards prescribing heparin differs with regard to whether to use it at all or not, and if yes, in what way (as a flush or in PN infusion), how often and how much. Boluses in children frequently contain 200–300 U of heparin, and for infants weighing less than 10 kg, a dose of 10 U/kg is frequently used [154] (LOE 2++).

In a meta-analysis (including mainly adult studies) evaluating the benefit of heparin prophylaxis in patients with CVCs, the risk of central venous thrombosis was significantly reduced [155] (LOE 1+).

Studies in the paediatric population did not demonstrate significant differences in catheter patency in groups of patients treated with heparin versus normal saline [156, 157] (LOE 1+); [158] (LOE 1–). However, all studies had a small sample size and thus not enough statistical power to draw definitive conclusions.

— There is no proven benefit of heparin for the prevention of thrombotic occlusion of CVCs **under regular use** in children. Therefore its routine use is not recommended. **LOE 1–**

- In adults flushing of CVCs **not in regular use** with 5–10 U/ml of heparinised saline once to twice weekly was useful in maintaining CVC patency and is recommended. **GOR D**
- Routine use of heparin has not been shown to be useful in prevention of complications related to peripherally placed percutaneous CVCs in neonates. **LOE 1–**

Skin Antisepsis and Hygiene

Recommendations

- Before insertion of an intravascular device and for post-insertion site care, clean skin should be disinfected. Application of 2% chlorhexidine is preferred, rather than 10% povidone iodine or 70% alcohol [159]. **GOR A**
- Antiseptic solution should remain on the insertion site and air-dry before catheter insertion or dressing application. **GOR D**
- Organic solvents (acetone, ether, etc.) should not to be applied to the skin before insertion of a catheter or during dressing changes. **GOR D**

Dressing Methods and Frequency of Dressing Changes

Statements and Recommendations

- Both, sterile gauze + tape and various transparent polyurethane film dressings can be used for catheter site care [160]. **GOR A**
- If the catheter site is bleeding or oozing, a gauze dressing is preferable to a transparent, semi-permeable dressing. **LOE 4**
- The catheter site dressing should be replaced when it becomes damp, loosened, or when inspection of the site is necessary. **GOR D**
- On short-term CVC sites dressings should be replaced every 2 days for gauze dressings and at least every 7 days for transparent dressings, except in those paediatric patients in which the risk of dislodging the catheter outweighs the benefit of changing the dressing. **GOR B**
- Topical antimicrobial ointments should not be used routinely at the insertion site as they may promote fungal infection, antimicrobial resistance and damage the surface of the catheters. **GOR D**
- With tunnelled catheters swimming is possible if the catheter is secured with water-resistant dressing [161]. **LOE 4**

Individualised versus Standard PN/Computer-Assisted Prescribing

Statement and Recommendations

— Standard PN solutions can be used for short periods of up to 2 weeks in many patients with adequate monitoring (table 11) and the scope for addition of deficient electrolytes and nutrients **(LOE 4)** if a range of standard regimens to suit different clinical conditions is available. **GOR D**

— Computer-assisted individual prescribing of PN is encouraged, since it can save time and improve the quality of nutritional care. **GOR B**

Monitoring

Table 11. Suggested assessment prior to ordering PN for infants and children depending on clinical status **(LOE 4)**

— Complete diet history	— Glucose
— Anthropometry (weight, height/length, head circumference)	— Calcium/phosphate
	— Albumin (or pre-albumin)
— Full blood count (including platelets and differential white count)	— Liver function tests
	— Cholesterol/triglycerides
— Electrolytes	— Urinary glucose and ketones
— Urea/creatinine	

These parameters should initially be assessed 2–3 times/week, and the frequency be consecutively reduced depending on the patients' clinical status and long-term goals. When PN extends beyond 3 months, trace elements, ferritin, folate, vitamin B_{12}, thyroid function, clotting, and fat-soluble vitamins are often measured.

Nutritional Assessment

Regular measurements of height, weight and head circumference with comparison to normal values for chronological age using percentile charts remain the most useful assessment tools for nutritional interventions [162] (LOE 4).

Subjective assessment must include a dietary record that focuses on nutritional history.

Weaning from PN

The following factors should be considered when introducing EN:

- Appropriate minimal enteral feeds should be given whenever possible to prevent gut atrophy [163] (LOE 3), encourage adaptation [164, 165] (LOE 3); [166, 167] (LOE 4), and reduce the risk of PN-associated liver disease [168] (LOE 3). In newborn infants with short gut expressed breast milk is the preferred nutrition. Breast milk should be given either fresh (in case of small bolus feeding) or pasteurised (in case of continuous feeding).
- Always make one change in treatment at a time to assess tolerance, e.g., when the volume of EN is increased, the concentration of the nutrition solution should remain constant.
- In severe intestinal failure feed volumes should be increased slowly, according to digestive tolerance.
- An experienced dietician/nutrition support team should be involved in the process.
- Central venous access should be maintained until the child can be fully fed enterally.
- Enteral feeding can be introduced as continuous EN over 4- to 24-hour periods, using a volumetric pump via an artificial feeding device. Some children can be weaned straight onto bolus feeds.
- Liquid EN can be given as bolus or sip feeds either orally or via an artificial feeding device, if tolerated.
- Children with a primary gastrointestinal disease causing intestinal failure usually require a specially formulated paediatric enteral feed when weaning.
- Children with rapid intestinal function recovery may be weaned straight onto normal food.

How to Wean

In children with more severe intestinal failure, enteral feeds may need to be introduced and increased as slowly as 1 ml/kg per 24 h. PN might be reduced by 5 ml/kg per 24 h every few days. Supplementary EN should generally be given undiluted at normal concentrations (GOR D). When EN is increased, PN should be reduced by similar or slightly greater amounts (GOR D). If a chosen weaning strategy fails it is worth trying again, but at a slower pace, e.g., with smaller rate increments.

Psycho-Social and Developmental Aspects of Feeding

Solids should be started at the usual recommended age for healthy infants when possible. When food is introduced, the aim is to encourage normal textures for age [169] (LOE 4). Even if the amount and range of foods are limited, introducing normal food will promote normal feeding behaviour.

Recommendation

— Whenever possible small volumes of oral feeds should be maintained. **GOR D**

Infusion Equipment and Inline Filters

PN solutions contain particulate matter [170] and biochemical interactions can lead to chemical precipitates and emulsion instability. PN solutions are also media for microbiological contamination. The routine use of inline filtration has been advocated and is considered mandatory.

Recommendations

— All PN solutions should be administered with accurate flow control. The infusion system should undergo regular visual inspection. Peripheral infusions should be checked frequently for signs of extravasation. The pump should have free flow prevention if opened during use, and have lockable settings. **GOR D**

— All PN solutions should be administered through a terminal filter. Lipid emulsion (or all-in-one mixes) should be passed through a membrane of pore size around 1.2–1.5 µm. Aqueous only solutions should be passed through a filter of 0.22 µm. **GOR D**

Nutrition Support Teams

Recommendation

— Supervision of PN patients necessitates a multidisciplinary nutritional support team as this is associated with decreased use of inappropriate PN, and decreased metabolic and catheter-related complications. **GOR D**

Age for safely commencing PN at home (HPN) depends on each individual condition. Most paediatric HPN programmes cater to children under 1 year of age and include babies under the age of 6 months [171, 172] (LOE 3). Patients eligible for HPN should be in a stable condition. This includes stability of the underlying disease, fluid and electrolyte requirements, and reliable central venous access.

Family suitability for HPN must be carefully assessed by a healthcare team member [173] (LOE 4) before a child's HPN programme is organised.

Statement and Recommendation

— HPN is usually less costly than hospital care. **LOE 2+**

— All children who depend on long-term PN should be discharged on HPN, if familial criteria are fulfilled. **GOR D**

Preparation of an HPN Paediatric Programme

Prior to discharge, parents must undergo structured training in all aspects of care and complications (table 12) [174, 175] (LOE 3); [176–178] (LOE 4). The structured teaching programme must have a written plan, including step-by-step instructions, and a method to record competence comprising theoretical and practical aspects.

Pumps

The main requirements for pump safety are: volumetric accuracy in a wide range of flow rates; no risk of sudden discontinuation of infusion (reliable battery); no risk of free flow; 'keep vein open' status; audible and written alarms (e.g. for air bubbles in line, empty container, occlusion, change in pressure, dose limit or low battery), and child proof [179] (LOE 4). Important for the quality of life are: simplicity to prime the set and clear air; pre-selection of infusion rates and of programmed stepwise increased and decreased flow rates at the onset and end of the infusion times; minimum false alarms; minimum motor noise, and minimum weight and volume with carrying handle and binding on i.v. poles.

— Flow control should be provided by a pump with free flow prevention, air alarm, occlusion alarm and lockable settings. **GOR D**

Nutrition Mixtures for Paediatric HPN

Recommendations

— The patient should be on a stable regime before starting PN. **GOR D**

— Standard PN mixtures are usually not suitable for long-term PN in infants and young children. Therefore, PN solutions providing macro- and micronutrients for paediatric HPN should be compounded according to individual patients needs. **GOR D**

— HPN delivery should be cyclic. A progressive increase and decrease in infusion rate should be considered to avoid hypo-/hyperglycaemia. **GOR D**

Organisation – Monitoring and Follow-Up

Recommendations

— Centres caring for infants and children on HPN must have adequate expertise and resources, including multidisciplinary nutrition support teams, trained and qualified to be responsible for use and prescription of HPN in children and a 24-hour telephone hotline. **GOR D**

— Paediatric HPN patients must be followed up by an experienced team on a regular basis (table 13). **GOR D**

Table 12. Parents' knowledge required before home discharge on HPN

Parents' knowledge	Handling	Catheter and line	Pump	Child
Current care	Hand washing technique	Flushing or heparinisation	Operation	Catheter exit site
	Preparation of sterile field	Initiation and termination of infusion	Maintenance	Temperature
	Drawing up solutions into syringe			
Emergency	Materials missing	Blockage of line	Alarms	Exit site infection
What to do?		Breakage/split catheter		Fever
Who to contact?		Air in the line		Digestive problem

Table 13. Clinical and biological monitoring in children on long-term HPN

Intervals	Clinical assessment	Other investigations
1–3 months	Weight	ALT, bilirubin, GGT, alkaline phosphatase
	Height	Blood chemistry, including Ca, P, Mg, urea, creatinine
	Clinical examination	Blood count
	Dietetic assessment	Clotting tests
		Urinary electrolytes (Ca, Na, K)
		Ferritin, zinc
		Thyroid function parameters
6 months to 1 year		Plasma vitamins A, E and D
		Liver and biliary tract ultrasonography
		Bone densitometry

Complications

Infection

Infection should be suspected if the child develops clinical signs such as fever (temperature >38.5°C or rise in temperature of >1°C), metabolic acidosis, thrombocytopenia or glucose instability.

Fungal CVC infection is an indication to remove the CVC. Persistent pyrexia with positive blood cultures after 48 h of appropriate antibiotics may be an indication to remove the CVC.

Recommendations

— PN fluids should be prepared in a suitable environment for aseptic compounding according to Good Pharmaceutical Manufacturing Practice. **GOR D**

— Amino acid/glucose infusion sets and extensions should be changed after no more than 72 h or as recommended by manufacturer. **GOR A**

— Lipid sets should be changed after no more than 24 h or as recommended by manufacturer. **GOR B**

— Carers should be taught about the signs of catheter-related sepsis (CRS). **GOR D**

— CVC blood cultures should be taken for any unexplained fever or other signs of CRS. **GOR D**

— Simultaneous peripheral blood cultures are generally only useful if a semi-quantitative or quantitative culture technique is used. **GOR D**

— For suspected CRS broad-spectrum i.v. antibiotics should be commenced promptly after taking CVC blood cultures, the choice of agents being based on local resistance patterns. Change to narrower-spectrum therapy should be practiced once the infecting micro-organism(s) has/have been identified. The duration of therapy should be guided by the organism identified. **GOR D**

— CVC complication rates should be audited continually, any change should be investigated and appropriate action taken. **GOR D**

Occlusion

Occlusion of the CVC can originate within the CVC lumen (blood, drug or PN fluid precipitate), in the vein (clot or fibrin sheath), external to the CVC due to the tip resting against a vein wall or due to external compression, e.g. clavicle, or patient positioning.

If mal-position or occlusion is suspected (e.g. inability to aspirate from catheter, increased infusion pressures), a chest X-ray should be performed to verify the catheter tip position [180] (LOE 3); [181] (LOE 4).

CVC occlusion can be treated with urokinase or alteplase for suspected blood deposits and ethyl alcohol or hydrochloric acid for suspected lipid or drug deposits [181] (LOE 4); [180, 182–189] (LOE 3). A combination of more than one treatment may be required. Catheter venography should be performed for persistent or recurrent occlusion [180, 181, 190] (LOE 4).

Recommendations

— Sodium chloride 0.9% should be used to flush the CVC between all therapies and heparin should be instilled at least weekly when the CVC is not in use. **GOR D**

— Terminal in-line filters should be used for all PN fluids. **GOR D**

— Occlusion of in-line filters should be investigated. **GOR D**

— Using the CVC for blood sampling should be avoided if possible. **GOR D**

— Leakage from the exit site, stiffness of the CVC or increased infusion pressures should be reported immediately to an experienced practitioner and appropriate investigations performed. **GOR D**

— CVC occlusion can be treated with urokinase or alteplase for suspected blood deposits and ethyl alcohol or hydrochloric acid for suspected lipid or drug deposits. **GOR D**

— Syringes less than 10 ml should not be routinely used on CVCs as they can generate very high internal pressures. **GOR D**

— Unblocking the CVC with a guide-wire is not recommended. **GOR D**

Central Venous Thrombosis and Pulmonary Embolism

Central venous thrombosis may result in facial swelling, prominent superficial veins or pain on commencing PN. Pulmonary embolism may present with chest pain, dyspnoea, haemoptysis, syncope, tachypnoea, tachycardia, sweating and fever. Small thrombi may be asymptomatic or have vague symptoms such as tiredness.

Central venous thrombosis and pulmonary embolism are associated with recurrent CVC infection, repeated CVC changes, proximal location of the CVC tip in the superior vena cava, frequent blood sampling, concentrated glucose solutions, chemotherapeutic agents, or may be idiopathic.

Removing the catheter should be considered, especially if infected [191] (LOE 3); [192, 193] (LOE 4). Vitamin K antagonists [194] (LOE 1/2); [195] (LOE 3) or low molecular weight heparins [196] (LOE 1/2) may reduce the risk of thrombo-embolism and may be given to patients on long-term PN with previous thrombo-embolism or at increased risk of thrombo-embolism.

Recommendations

— Symptoms or signs of thrombo-embolism should be reported immediately to an experienced practitioner and appropriate investigations performed. **GOR D**

— Acute symptomatic thrombosis can be treated with thrombolytic agents or anticoagulation. **GOR D**

Accidental Removal or Damage

Dressings should stay in situ as per surgeons' instructions unless they become damp, soiled, loosened or there is swelling, bleeding and/or leakage from the CVC exit site and the dressing prevents observation.

Recommendations

— CVCs should be securely taped to the body to prevent accidental removal, traction or damage. **GOR D**

— Postoperative dressings should be secure but allow observation of the exit site and easy dressing removal. **GOR D**

- Any damage to the CVC should be reported immediately to an experienced practitioner and appropriate repairs performed promptly. **GOR D**
- Luer lock connectors should be used to reduce the risk of accidental leakage and haemorrhage. **GOR D**
- Clamps should be available at all times to prevent bleeding from a damaged CVC. **GOR D**
- Children (as soon as they are aware) and all carers should be educated about the safety of the CVC. **GOR D**

Compatibility

PN in paediatrics can be admixed into '2 in 1' or '3 in 1' admixtures. A '2 in 1' admixture is one that contains amino acids, carbohydrates and electrolytes in a single container with lipid emulsion kept in a separate container. A '3 in 1' admixture has all the components including lipid in a single container. With up to 100 chemical species present in an admixture, enormous potential for interaction exists. Even in validated admixture formulations there may still be variability through factors such as the variation in pH between different batches of glucose due to decomposition during autoclaving [197] (LOE 4), and changes in trace element profiles due to adsorption onto, or leaching from, admixture containers and tubing [198–200] (LOE 3).

Using a '2 in 1' admixture means that the lipid emulsion is infused 'separately' but in practice this usually means into the same infusion line, through a 'Y' connector. This approach does not ensure stability [201, 202] (LOE 3).

Addition of heparin to admixtures, even where validated, carries a small risk of emulsion instability occurring with individual batches of heparin [203] (LOE 4).

Recommendations

- PN should be administered wherever possible using an admixture formulation validated by a licensed manufacturer or suitably qualified institution. **GOR D**

- A matrix table should be sought from the supplier of the formulation detailing permissible limits for additions of electrolytes and other additives. **GOR D**
- Alternative ingredients should not be substituted without expert advice or repeat validation. **GOR D**
- Phosphate should be added in an organic-bound form to prevent the risk of calcium-phosphate precipitation. **GOR D**
- If inorganic phosphate is used, stability matrices and order of mixing must be strictly adhered to and occasional precipitates may still occur. **GOR D**
- Use of '2 in 1' admixtures with Y-site addition of lipids should be fully validated by the manufacturer or accredited laboratory or the lipid infused through an alternative line. **GOR D**
- As there are risks associated with instability of regimens, PN admixtures should be administered through a terminal filter [204]. **GOR D**

Drug Interactions

Recommendations

- Mixing of medications with PN in administration lines should be avoided unless validated by the manufacturer or accredited laboratory. **GOR D**
- Medications known to affect plasma protein binding of bilirubin should be avoided in parenterally fed newborn patients with severe hyperbilirubinaemia. **GOR D**

Metabolic Bone Disease

PN-related metabolic bone disease with a decrease in bone mineral density, osteoporosis, pain and fractures has been described in adults on long-term PN. Few data exist in children, although its occurrence has been reported in children weaned from long-term PN [205–207] (LOE 3). The cause of metabolic bone disease is probably multifactorial including both underlying disease and PN-related mechanisms: excess vitamin D, phosphorus, nitrogen and energy imbalance, excess amino acids and aluminium contamination [208] (LOE 3).

— In children on HPN, regular measurements of urinary calcium, plasma calcium, phosphorus, parathyroid hormone and vitamin D concentrations and serum alkaline phosphatase activity should be performed. **GOR D**

— Aluminium contamination of PN solutions provided to patients receiving long-term PN should be kept to a minimum (avoid glass vials and certain minerals and trace elements known to have high aluminium content). **GOR D**

— Regular assessment of bone mineralisation should be performed. **GOR D**

Hepatobiliary Complications of PN

The pathogenesis of PN-associated liver disease is not completely understood [209] (LOE 3); [210] (LOE 4). It probably results from the interaction of many factors related to the underlying disease, infectious episodes and components of the PN solution [1, 211, 212] (LOE 4).

— Liver disease should be prevented by reducing patient-related and PN-related risk factors. **GOR D**

— Provide maximal tolerated EN even if minimal residual gut function. **GOR A**

— Commence cyclical PN as soon as possible. **GOR C**

— Consider and treat intraluminal bacterial overgrowth. **GOR D**

— Consider reducing or stopping i.v. lipids temporarily if conjugated bilirubin steadily increases with no other explanation. **GOR D**

— If transaminases, alkaline phosphatase or conjugated bilirubin continue to increase consider commencing ursodeoxycholic acid. **GOR D**

— Early referral to an experienced paediatric liver and intestinal transplant centre for further assessment is recommended in infants/children with poor prognosis or if on PN for >3 months and serum bilirubin >50 μmol/l, platelet count <100, PT >15 sec, PTT >40 sec or hepatic fibrosis. **GOR D**

References

1 Koletzko B, Goulet O, Hunt J, Krohn K, Shamir R: 1. Guidelines on Paediatric Parenteral Nutrition of the European Society of Paediatric Gastroenterology, Hepatology and Nutrition (ESPGHAN) and the European Society for Clinical Nutrition and Metabolism (ESPEN), Supported by the European Society of Paediatric Research (ESPR). J Pediatr Gastroenterol Nutr 2005;41(suppl 2):S1–S87.

2 Elia M: Changing concepts of nutrient requirements in disease: implications for artificial nutritional support. Lancet 1995;345:1279–1284.

3 Sheldon GF, Peterson SR, Sanders R: Hepatic dysfunction during hyperalimentation. Arch Surg 1978;113:504–508.

4 Torun B, Chew F: Protein-energy malnutrition; in Shils M, Shike M, Olson J (eds): Modern Nutrition in Health and Disease. Baltimore, Williams & Wilkins, 1999, pp 963–988.

5 Koretz RL, Lipman TO, Klein S: AGA technical review on parenteral nutrition. Gastroenterology 2001;121:970–1001.

6 Thureen PJ, Hay WW Jr: Intravenous nutrition and postnatal growth of the micropremie. Clin Perinatol 2000;27:197–219.

7 Lloyd DA: Energy requirements of surgical newborn infants receiving parenteral nutrition. Nutrition 1998;14:101–104.

8 Powis MR, Smith K, Rennie M, Halliday D, Pierro A: Effect of major abdominal operations on energy and protein metabolism in infants and children. J Pediatr Surg 1998;33:49–53.

9 Bresson JL, Bader B, Rocchiccioli F, Mariotti A, Ricour C, Sachs C, et al: Protein-metabolism kinetics and energy-substrate utilization in infants fed parenteral solutions with different glucose-fat ratios. Am J Clin Nutr 1991;54:370–376.

10 Pierro A, Carnielli V, Filler RM, Smith J, Heim T: Metabolism of intravenous fat emulsion in the surgical newborn. J Pediatr Surg 1989;24:95–101.

11 Cooke RJ, Zee P, Yeh YY: Essential fatty acid status of the premature infant during short-term fat-free parenteral nutrition. J Pediatr Gastroenterol Nutr 1984;3:446–449.

12 Friedman Z, Danon A, Stahlman MT, Oates JA: Rapid onset of essential fatty acid deficiency in the newborn. Pediatrics 1976;58:640–649.

13 Lee EJ, Simmer K, Gibson RA: Essential fatty acid deficiency in parenterally fed preterm infants. J Paediatr Child Health 1993;29:51–55.

14 Brans YW, Andrew DS, Carrillo DW, Dutton EP, Menchaca EM, Puleo-Scheppke BA: Tolerance of fat emulsions in very-low-birth-weight neonates. Am J Dis Child 1988;142:145–152.

15 Hilliard JL, Shannon DL, Hunter MA, Brans YW: Plasma lipid levels in preterm neonates receiving parenteral fat emulsions. Arch Dis Child 1983;58:29–33.

16 Kao LC, Cheng MH, Warburton D: Triglycerides, free fatty acids, free fatty acids/albumin molar ratio, and cholesterol levels in serum of neonates receiving long-term lipid infusions: controlled trial of continuous and intermittent regimens. J Pediatr 1984;104:429–435.

17 Brans YW, Andrew DS, Carrillo DW, Dutton EB, Menchaca EM, Puelo-Scheppke BA: Tolerance of fat emulsions in very low birthweight neonates: effect of birthweight on plasma lipid concentrations. Am J Perinatol 1990;7:114–117.

18   Brans YW, Dutton EB, Andrew DS, Menchaca EM, West DL: Fat emulsion tolerance in very low birth weight neonates: effect on diffusion of oxygen in the lungs and on blood pH. Pediatrics 1986;78:79–84.

19   Dhanireddy R, Hamosh M, Sivasubramanian KN, Chowdhry P, Scanlon JW, Hamosh P: Postheparin lipolytic activity and Intralipid clearance in very low-birth-weight infants. J Pediatr 1981;98:617–622.

20   Spear ML, Stahl GE, Hamosh M, McNelis WG, Richardson LL, Spence V, et al: Effect of heparin dose and infusion rate on lipid clearance and bilirubin binding in premature infants receiving intravenous fat emulsions. J Pediatr 1988;112:94–98.

21   Berkow SE, Spear ML, Stahl GE, Gutman A, Polin RA, Pereira GR, et al: Total parenteral nutrition with intralipid in premature infants receiving TPN with heparin: effect on plasma lipolytic enzymes, lipids, and glucose. J Pediatr Gastroenterol Nutr 1987;6:581–588.

22   Peterson J, Bihain BE, Bengtsson-Olivecrona G, Deckelbaum RJ, Carpentier YA, Olivecrona T: Fatty acid control of lipoprotein lipase: a link between energy metabolism and lipid transport. Proc Natl Acad Sci USA 1990;87:909–913.

23   Shulman RJ, Phillips S: Parenteral nutrition in infants and children. J Pediatr Gastroenterol Nutr 2003;36:587–607.

24   Connelly PW, Maguire GF, Vezina C, Hegele RA, Kuksis A: Kinetics of lipolysis of very low density lipoproteins by lipoprotein lipase. Importance of particle number and noncompetitive inhibition by particles with low triglyceride content. J Biol Chem 1994;269:20554–20560.

25   Deckelbaum RJ: Intravenous lipid emulsions in pediatrics: time for a change? J Pediatr Gastroenterol Nutr 2003;37:112–114.

26   Cairns PA, Stalker DJ: Carnitine supplementation of parenterally fed neonates. Cochrane Database Syst Rev 2000;(4):CD000950.

27   Goel R, Hamosh M, Stahl GE, Henderson TR, Spear ML, Hamosh P: Plasma lecithin: cholesterol acyltransferase and plasma lipolytic activity in preterm infants given total parenteral nutrition with 10% or 20% Intralipid. Acta Paediatr 1995;84:1060–1064.

28   Haumont D, Deckelbaum RJ, Richelle M, Dahlan W, Coussaert E, Bihain BE, et al: Plasma lipid and plasma lipoprotein concentrations in low birth weight infants given parenteral nutrition with twenty or ten percent lipid emulsion. J Pediatr 1989;115:787–793.

29   Gilbertson N, Kovar IZ, Cox DJ, Crowe L, Palmer NT: Introduction of intravenous lipid administration on the first day of life in the very low birth weight neonate. J Pediatr 1991;119:615–623.

30   Fox GF, Wilson DC: Effect of early vs. late introduction of intravenous lipid to preterm infants on death and chronic lung disease (CLD) – results of meta-analyses. Pediatr Res 1998;43:214A.

31   Sosenko IR, Rodriguez-Pierce M, Bancalari E: Effect of early initiation of intravenous lipid administration on the incidence and severity of chronic lung disease in premature infants. J Pediatr 1993;123:975–982.

32   Neuzil J, Darlow BA, Inder TE, Sluis KB, Winterbourn CC, Stocker R: Oxidation of parenteral lipid emulsion by ambient and phototherapy lights: potential toxicity of routine parenteral feeding. J Pediatr 1995;126:785–790.

33 Brans YW, Ritter DA, Kenny JD, Andrew DS, Dutton EB, Carrillo DW: Influence of intravenous fat emulsion on serum bilirubin in very low birthweight neonates. Arch Dis Child 1987; 62:156–160.

34 Rubin M, Naor N, Sirota L, Moser A, Pakula R, Harell D, et al: Are bilirubin and plasma lipid profiles of premature infants dependent on the lipid emulsion infused? J Pediatr Gastroenterol Nutr 1995;21:25–30.

35 Schmidt-Sommerfeld E, Penn D: Carnitine and total parenteral nutrition of the neonate. Biol Neonate 1990;58(suppl 1):81–88.

36 Robin AP, Carpentier YA, Askanazi J, Nordenstrom J, Kinney JM: Metabolic consequences of hypercaloric glucose infusions. Acta Chir Belg 1981;80:133–140.

37 Elwyn DH, Askanazi J, Kinney JM, Gump FE: Kinetics of energy substrates. Acta Chir Scand Suppl 1981;507:209–219.

38 Talpers SS, Romberger DJ, Bunce SB, Pingleton SK: Nutritionally associated increased carbon dioxide production. Excess total calories vs high proportion of carbohydrate calories. Chest 1992;102:551–555.

39 Askanazi J, Weissman C, LaSala PA, Milic-Emili J, Kinney JM: Effect of protein intake on ventilatory drive. Anesthesiology 1984;60:106–110.

40 Rodriguez JL, Askanazi J, Weissman C, Hensle TW, Rosenbaum SH, Kinney JM: Ventilatory and metabolic effects of glucose infusions. Chest 1985;88:512–518.

41 Kalhan SC, Kilic I: Carbohydrate as nutrient in the infant and child: range of acceptable intake. Eur J Clin Nutr 1999;53(suppl 1):S94–S100.

42 Denne SC, Karn CA, Wang J, Liechty EA: Effect of intravenous glucose and lipid on proteolysis and glucose production in normal newborns. Am J Physiol 1995;269:E361–E367.

43 Sunehag AL, Haymond MW, Schanler RJ, Reeds PJ, Bier DM: Gluconeogenesis in very low birth weight infants receiving total parenteral nutrition. Diabetes 1999;48:791–800.

44 Lafeber HN, Sulkers EJ, Chapman TE, Sauer PJ: Glucose production and oxidation in preterm infants during total parenteral nutrition. Pediatr Res 1990;28:153–157.

45 Forsyth JS, Crighton A: Low birthweight infants and total parenteral nutrition immediately after birth. I. Energy expenditure and respiratory quotient of ventilated and non-ventilated infants. Arch Dis Child Fetal Neonatal Ed 1995;73:F4–F7.

46 Sauer PJ, Van Aerde JE, Pencharz PB, Smith JM, Swyer PR: Glucose oxidation rates in newborn infants measured with indirect calorimetry and [U-^{13}C]glucose. Clin Sci (Lond) 1986; 70:587–593.

47 Jones MO, Pierro A, Hammond P, Nunn A, Lloyd DA: Glucose utilization in the surgical newborn infant receiving total parenteral nutrition. J Pediatr Surg 1993;28:1121–1125.

48 Nose O, Tipton JR, Ament ME, Yabuuchi H: Effect of the energy source on changes in energy expenditure, respiratory quotient, and nitrogen balance during total parenteral nutrition in children. Pediatr Res 1987;21:538–541.

49 Sheridan RL, Yu YM, Prelack K, Young VR, Burke JF, Tompkins RG: Maximal parenteral glucose oxidation in hypermetabolic young children: a stable isotope study. JPEN J Parenter Enteral Nutr 1998;22:212–216.

50 Van den Berghe G: Beyond diabetes: saving lives with insulin in the ICU. Int J Obes Relat Metab Disord 2002;26(suppl 3):S3–S8.

51 Modi N: Development of renal function. Br Med Bull 1988;44:935–956.

52 Coulthard MG, Hey EN: Effect of varying water intake on renal function in healthy preterm babies. Arch Dis Child 1985;60:614–620.

53 Bell EF, Acarregui MJ: Restricted versus liberal water intake for preventing morbidity and mortality in preterm infants. Cochrane Database Syst Rev 2001;(3):CD000503.

54 Hartnoll G, Betremieux P, Modi N: Randomised controlled trial of postnatal sodium supplementation on body composition in 25 to 30 week gestational age infants. Arch Dis Child Fetal Neonatal Ed 2000;82:F24–F28.

55 Al-Dahhan J, Haycock GB, Nichol B, Chantler C, Stimmler L: Sodium homeostasis in term and preterm neonates. III. Effect of salt supplementation. Arch Dis Child 1984;59:945–950.

56 Burcar PJ, Norenberg MD, Yarnell PR: Hyponatremia and central pontine myelinolysis. Neurology 1977;27:223–226.

57 Adamkin DH: Issues in the nutritional support of the ventilated baby. Clin Perinatol 1998; 25:79–96.

58 Winters R: Maintenance Fluid Therapy. The Body Fluids in Pediatrics. Boston, Little Brown, 1973.

59 Sinclair JC: Metabolic rate and temperature control; in Smith CA, Nelson N (eds): The Physiology of the Newborn Infant. Springfield, Thomas, 1976, pp 354–415.

60 Sosulski R, Polin RA, Baumgart S: Respiratory water loss and heat balance in intubated infants receiving humidified air. J Pediatr 1983;103:307–310.

61 Weil WB, Bailie MD: Fluid and Electrolyte Metabolism in Infants and Children. A Unified Approach. New York, Grune & Station, 1977.

62 Burns DL, Pomposelli JJ: Toxicity of parenteral iron dextran therapy. Kidney Int Suppl 1999;69:S119–S124.

63 Reed MD, Bertino JS Jr, Halpin TC Jr: Use of intravenous iron dextran injection in children receiving total parenteral nutrition. Am J Dis Child 1981;135:829–831.

64 Vaughan LM, Small C, Plunkett V: Incompatibility of iron dextran and a total nutrient admixture. Am J Hosp Pharm 1990;47:1745–1746.

65 Allwood MC, Kearney MC: Compatibility and stability of additives in parenteral nutrition admixtures. Nutrition 1998;14:697–706.

66 Van Gossum A, Neve J: Trace element deficiency and toxicity. Curr Opin Clin Nutr Metab Care 1998;1:499–507.

67 Leung FY, Galbraith LV: Elevated serum chromium in patients on total parenteral nutrition and the ionic species of contaminant chromium. Biol Trace Elem Res 1995;50:221–228.

68 Greene HL, Hambidge KM, Schanler R, Tsang RC: Guidelines for the use of vitamins, trace elements, calcium, magnesium, and phosphorus in infants and children receiving total parenteral nutrition: report of the Subcommittee on Pediatric Parenteral Nutrient Requirements from the Committee on Clinical Practice Issues of the American Society for Clinical Nutrition. Am J Clin Nutr 1988;48:1324–1342.

69 Schanler RJ, Shulman RJ, Prestridge LL: Parenteral nutrient needs of very low birth weight infants. J Pediatr 1994;125:961–968.

70 Committee on Nutrition AAoP: Nutritional needs of preterm infants; in Kleinman RE (ed): Pediatric Nutrition Handbook. Elk Grove Village, American Academy of Pediatrics, 1998, pp 55–88.

71 Moukarzel AA, Song MK, Buchman AL, Vargas J, Guss W, McDiarmid S, et al: Excessive chromium intake in children receiving total parenteral nutrition. Lancet 1992;339:385–388.

72 Hak EB, Storm MC, Helms RA: Chromium and zinc contamination of parenteral nutrient solution components commonly used in infants and children. Am J Health Syst Pharm 1998;55:150–154.

73 Fell JM, Reynolds AP, Meadows N, Khan K, Long SG, Quaghebeur G, et al: Manganese toxicity in children receiving long-term parenteral nutrition. Lancet 1996;347:1218–1221.

74 Cunningham JJ, Leffell M, Harmatz P: Burn severity, copper dose, and plasma ceruloplasmin in burned children during total parenteral nutrition. Nutrition 1993;9:329–332.

75 Cunningham JJ, Lydon MK, Briggs SE, DeCheke M: Zinc and copper status of severely burned children during TPN. J Am Coll Nutr 1991;10:57–62.

76 Reynolds AP, Kiely E, Meadows N: Manganese in long term paediatric parenteral nutrition. Arch Dis Child 1994;71:527–528.

77 Kelly DA: Liver complications of pediatric parenteral nutrition – epidemiology. Nutrition 1998;14:153–157.

78 Fok TF, Chui KK, Cheung R, Ng PC, Cheung KL, Hjelm M: Manganese intake and cholestatic jaundice in neonates receiving parenteral nutrition: a randomized controlled study. Acta Paediatr 2001;90:1009–1015.

79 Masumoto K, Suita S, Taguchi T, Yamanouchi T, Nagano M, Ogita K, et al: Manganese intoxication during intermittent parenteral nutrition: report of two cases. JPEN J Parenter Enteral Nutr 2001;25:95–99.

80 Puntis JW: Nutritional support at home and in the community. Arch Dis Child 2001;84:295–298.

81 Ono J, Harada K, Kodaka R, Sakurai K, Tajiri H, Takagi Y, et al: Manganese deposition in the brain during long-term total parenteral nutrition. JPEN J Parenter Enteral Nutr 1995;19:310–312.

82 Kafritsa Y, Fell J, Long S, Bynevelt M, Taylor W, Milla P: Long-term outcome of brain manganese deposition in patients on home parenteral nutrition. Arch Dis Child 1998;79:263–265.

83 Komaki H, Maisawa S, Sugai K, Kobayashi Y, Hashimoto T: Tremor and seizures associated with chronic manganese intoxication. Brain Dev 1999;21:122–124.

84 Terada A, Nakada M, Nakada K, Yamate N, Tanaka Y, Yoshida M, et al: Selenium administration to a ten-year-old patient receiving long-term total parenteral nutrition (TPN) – changes in selenium concentration in the blood and hair. J Trace Elem Med Biol 1996;10:1–5.

85 Daniels L, Gibson R, Simmer K: Randomised clinical trial of parenteral selenium supplementation in preterm infants. Arch Dis Child Fetal Neonatal Ed 1996;74:F158–F164.

86 Klinger G, Shamir R, Singer P, Diamond EM, Josefsberg Z, Sirota L: Parenteral selenium supplementation in extremely low birth weight infants: inadequate dosage but no correlation with hypothyroidism. J Perinatol 1999;19:568–572.

87 Friel JK, Andrews WL: Zinc requirement of premature infants. Nutrition 1994;10:63–65.

88 Leung FY: Trace elements in parenteral micronutrition. Clin Biochem 1995;28:561–566.

89   Dunham B, Marcuard S, Khazanie PG, Meade G, Craft T, Nichols K: The solubility of calcium and phosphorus in neonatal total parenteral nutrition solutions. JPEN J Parenter Enteral Nutr 1991;15:608–611.

90   Fitzgerald KA, MacKay MW: Calcium and phosphate solubility in neonatal parenteral nutrient solutions containing TrophAmine. Am J Hosp Pharm 1986;43:88–93.

91   Poole RL, Rupp CA, Kerner JA Jr: Calcium and phosphorus in neonatal parenteral nutrition solutions. JPEN J Parenter Enteral Nutr 1983;7:358–360.

92   Venkataraman PS, Brissie EO Jr, Tsang RC: Stability of calcium and phosphorus in neonatal parenteral nutrition solutions. J Pediatr Gastroenterol Nutr 1983;2:640–643.

93   Colonna F, Candusso M, de Vonderweid U, Marinoni S, Gazzola AM: Calcium and phosphorus balance in very low birth weight babies on total parenteral nutrition. Clin Nutr 1990;9: 89–95.

94   Costello I, Powell C, Williams AF: Sodium glycerophosphate in the treatment of neonatal hypophosphataemia. Arch Dis Child Fetal Neonatal Ed 1995;73:F44–F45.

95   Devlieger H, Meyers Y, Willems L, de Zegher F, Van Lierde S, Proesmans W, et al: Calcium and phosphorus retention in the preterm infant during total parenteral nutrition. A comparative randomised study between organic and inorganic phosphate as a source of phosphorus. Clin Nutr 1993;12:277–281.

96   Draper HH, Yuen DE, Whyte RK: Calcium glycerophosphate as a source of calcium and phosphorus in total parenteral nutrition solutions. JPEN J Parenter Enteral Nutr 1991;15:176–180.

97   Hanning RM, Atkinson SA, Whyte RK: Efficacy of calcium glycerophosphate vs conventional mineral salts for total parenteral nutrition in low-birth-weight infants: a randomized clinical trial. Am J Clin Nutr 1991;54:903–908.

98   Hanning RM, Mitchell MK, Atkinson SA: In vitro solubility of calcium glycerophosphate versus conventional mineral salts in pediatric parenteral nutrition solutions. J Pediatr Gastroenterol Nutr 1989;9:67–72.

99   Prinzivalli M, Ceccarelli S: Sodium D-fructose-1,6-diphosphate vs. sodium monohydrogen phosphate in total parenteral nutrition: a comparative in vitro assessment of calcium phosphate compatibility. JPEN J Parenter Enteral Nutr 1999;23:326–332.

100 Raupp P, von Kries R, Pfahl HG, Manz F: Glycero- vs glucose-phosphate in parenteral nutrition of premature infants: a comparative in vitro evaluation of calcium/phosphorus compatibility. JPEN J Parenter Enteral Nutr 1991;15:469–473.

101 Ronchera-Oms CL, Jimenez NV, Peidro J: Stability of parenteral nutrition admixtures containing organic phosphates. Clin Nutr 1995;14:373–380.

102 Baessler KH, Hassinger W: Die Eignung von DL-Glyzerin-3-phosphat zur parenteralen Substitution von anorganischem Phosphat. Infusionstherapie 1976;3:138–142.

103 Pohlandt F: Prevention of postnatal bone demineralization in very low-birth-weight infants by individually monitored supplementation with calcium and phosphorus. Pediatr Res 1994;35:125–129.

104 Leitch I: The determination of the calcium requirements: a re-examination. Nutr Abstr Rev Ser Hum Exp 1937;6:553–578.

105 Leitch I, Aitken FC: The estimation of calcium requirement: a re-examination. Nutr Abstr Rev Ser Hum Exp 1959;29:393–411.

106 Ehrenkranz RA: Iron, folic acid and vitamin B_{12}; in Tsang RC, Lucas A, Uauy RD, Zlotkin S (eds): Nutritional Needs of the Preterm Infant. Baltimore, Williams & Wilkins, 1993, pp 177–194.

107 Greer FR: Vitamin metabolism and requirements in the micropremie. Clin Perinatol 2000;27:95–118, vi.

108 Baeckert PA, Greene HL, Fritz I, Oelberg DG, Adcock EW: Vitamin concentrations in very low birth weight infants given vitamins intravenously in a lipid emulsion: measurement of vitamins A, D, and E and riboflavin. J Pediatr 1988;113:1057–1065.

109 Inder TE, Carr AC, Winterbourn CC, Austin NC, Darlow BA: Vitamin A and E status in very low birth weight infants: development of an improved parenteral delivery system. J Pediatr 1995;126:128–131.

110 Werkman SH, Peeples JM, Cooke RJ, Tolley EA, Carlson SE: Effect of vitamin A supplementation of intravenous lipids on early vitamin A intake and status of premature infants. Am J Clin Nutr 1994;59:586–592.

111 Schwalbe P, Buttner P, Elmadfa I: Development of vitamin-E-status of premature infants after intravenous application of all-rac-alpha-tocopheryl acetate. Int J Vitam Nutr Res 1992;62:9–14.

112 Gross S: Vitamin E; in Tsang RC, Lucas A, Uauy RD, Zlotkin S (eds): Nutritional Needs of the Preterm Infant. Baltimore: Williams & Wilkins, 1993, pp 101–109.

113 Sokol RJ: Vitamin E toxicity. Pediatrics 1984;74:564–569.

114 Koo WW, Tsang RC, Succop P, Krug-Wispe SK, Babcock D, Oestreich AE: Minimal vitamin D and high calcium and phosphorus needs of preterm infants receiving parenteral nutrition. J Pediatr Gastroenterol Nutr 1989;8:225–233.

115 American Academy of Pediatrics: Nutritional Needs of Preterm Infants. Pediatric Nutrition Handbook. Elk Grove Village, American Academy of Pediatrics, 1998, pp 55–87.

116 Greene HL, Smith R, Pollack P, Murrell J, Caudill M, Swift L: Intravenous vitamins for very-low-birth-weight infants. J Am Coll Nutr 1991;10:281–288.

117 Porcelli PJ, Adcock EW, DelPaggio D, Swift LL, Greene HL: Plasma and urine riboflavin and pyridoxine concentrations in enterally fed very-low-birth-weight neonates. J Pediatr Gastroenterol Nutr 1996;23:141–146.

118 Lange R, Erhard J, Eigler FW, Roll C: Lactic acidosis from thiamine deficiency during parenteral nutrition in a two-year-old boy. Eur J Pediatr Surg 1992;2:241–244.

119 Friel JK, Bessie JC, Belkhode SL, Edgecombe C, Steele-Rodway M, Downton G, et al: Thiamine, riboflavin, pyridoxine, and vitamin C status in premature infants receiving parenteral and enteral nutrition. J Pediatr Gastroenterol Nutr 2001;33:64–69.

120 Silvers KM, Sluis KB, Darlow BA, McGill F, Stocker R, Winterbourn CC: Limiting light-induced lipid peroxidation and vitamin loss in infant parenteral nutrition by adding multivitamin preparations to Intralipid. Acta Paediatr 2001;90:242–249.

121 Greer FR: Vitamin K; in Tsang RC, Lucas A, Uauy RD, Zlotkin S (eds): Nutritional Needs of the Preterm Infant. Baltimore, Williams & Wilkins, 1993, pp 111–120.

122 Koo WW, Tsang RC: Calcium, magnesium, phosphorus and vitamin D; in Tsang RC, Lucas A, Uauy RD, Zlotkin S (eds): Nutritional Needs of the Preterm Infant. Baltimore, Williams & Wilkins, 1993, pp 135–175.

123 Shenai JP: Vitamin A; in Tsang RC, Lucas A, Uauy RD, Zlotkin S (eds): Nutritional Needs of the Preterm Infant. Baltimore, Williams & Wilkins, 1993, pp 87–100.

124 Bass WT, Malati N, Castle MC, White LE: Evidence for the safety of ascorbic acid administration to the premature infant. Am J Perinatol 1998;15:133–140.

125 Greene HL, Smith LJ: Water-soluble vitamins: C, B1, B12, B6, niacin, pantothenic acid, and biotin; in Tsang RC, Lucas A, Uauy RD, Zlotkin S (eds): Nutritional Needs of the Preterm Infant. Baltimore, Williams & Wilkins, 1993, pp 121–133.

126 Gazitua R, Wilson K, Bistrian BR, Blackburn GL: Factors determining peripheral vein tolerance to amino acid infusions. Arch Surg 1979;114:897–900.

127 Sheth NK, Franson TR, Rose HD, Buckmire FL, Cooper JA, Sohnle PG: Colonization of bacteria on polyvinyl chloride and Teflon intravascular catheters in hospitalized patients. J Clin Microbiol 1983;18:1061–1063.

128 Sank A, Chalabian-Baliozian J, Ertl D, Sherman R, Nimni M, Tuan TL: Cellular responses to silicone and polyurethane prosthetic surfaces. J Surg Res 1993;54:12–20.

129 Polderman KH, Girbes AJ: Central venous catheter use. Part 1: mechanical complications. Intensive Care Med 2002;28:1–17.

130 Venkataraman ST, Thompson AE, Orr RA: Femoral vascular catheterization in critically ill infants and children. Clin Pediatr (Phila) 1997;36:311–319.

131 Sovinz P, Urban C, Lackner H, Kerbl R, Schwinger W, Dornbusch H: Tunneled femoral central venous catheters in children with cancer. Pediatrics 2001;107:E104.

132 Murai DT: Are femoral Broviac catheters effective and safe? A prospective comparison of femoral and jugular venous broviac catheters in newborn infants. Chest 2002;121:1527–1530.

133 Stenzel JP, Green TP, Fuhrman BP, Carlson PE, Marchessault RP: Percutaneous femoral venous catheterizations: a prospective study of complications. J Pediatr 1989;114:411–415.

134 Goldstein AM, Weber JM, Sheridan RL: Femoral venous access is safe in burned children: an analysis of 224 catheters. J Pediatr 1997;130:442–446.

135 Chen KB: Clinical experience of percutaneous femoral venous catheterization in critically ill preterm infants less than 1,000 grams. Anesthesiology 2001;95:637–639.

136 Wardle SP, Kelsall AW, Yoxall CW, Subhedar NV: Percutaneous femoral arterial and venous catheterisation during neonatal intensive care. Arch Dis Child Fetal Neonatal Ed 2001;85: F119–F122.

137 Alderson PJ, Burrows FA, Stemp LI, Holtby HM: Use of ultrasound to evaluate internal jugular vein anatomy and to facilitate central venous cannulation in paediatric patients. Br J Anaesth 1993;70:145–148.

138 Fallat ME, Gallinaro RN, Stover BH, Wilkerson S, Goldsmith LJ: Central venous catheter bloodstream infections in the neonatal intensive care unit. J Pediatr Surg 1998;33:1383–1387.

139 Shaul DB, Scheer B, Rokhsar S, Jones VA, Chan LS, Boody BA, et al: Risk factors for early infection of central venous catheters in pediatric patients. J Am Coll Surg 1998;186:654–658.

140 Fletcher MA, Brown DR, Landers S, Seguin J: Umbilical arterial catheter use: report of an audit conducted by the Study Group for Complications of Perinatal Care. Am J Perinatol 1994;11:94–99.

141 Boo NY, Wong NC, Zulkifli SS, Lye MS: Risk factors associated with umbilical vascular catheter-associated thrombosis in newborn infants. J Paediatr Child Health 1999;35:460–465.

142 Seguin J, Fletcher MA, Landers S, Brown D, Macpherson T: Umbilical venous catheterizations: audit by the Study Group for Complications of Perinatal Care. Am J Perinatol 1994; 11:67–70.

143 Loisel DB, Smith MM, MacDonald MG, Martin GR: Intravenous access in newborn infants: impact of extended umbilical venous catheter use on requirement for peripheral venous lines. J Perinatol 1996;16:461–466.

144 Barrington KJ: Umbilical artery catheters in the newborn: effects of position of the catheter tip. Cochrane Database Syst Rev 2000;(2):CD000505.

145 Eyer S, Brummitt C, Crossley K, Siegel R, Cerra F: Catheter-related sepsis: prospective, randomized study of three methods of long-term catheter maintenance. Crit Care Med 1990; 18:1073–1079.

146 Cobb DK, High KP, Sawyer RG, Sable CA, Adams RB, Lindley DA, et al: A controlled trial of scheduled replacement of central venous and pulmonary-artery catheters. N Engl J Med 1992;327:1062–1068.

147 Cook D, Randolph A, Kernerman P, Cupido C, King D, Soukup C, et al: Central venous catheter replacement strategies: a systematic review of the literature. Crit Care Med 1997;25:1417–1424.

148 Apelgren KN: Triple lumen catheters. Technological advance or setback? Am Surg 1987;53:113–116.

149 Yeung C, May J, Hughes R: Infection rate for single lumen v triple lumen subclavian catheters. Infect Control Hosp Epidemiol 1988;9:154–158.

150 Lagro SW, Verdonck LF, Borel Rinkes IH, Dekker AW: No effect of nadroparin prophylaxis in the prevention of central venous catheter (CVC)-associated thrombosis in bone marrow transplant recipients. Bone Marrow Transplant 2000;26:1103–1106.

151 Pemberton LB, Lyman B, Lander V, Covinsky J: Sepsis from triple- vs single-lumen catheters during total parenteral nutrition in surgical or critically ill patients. Arch Surg 1986;121:591–594.

152 Hilton E, Haslett TM, Borenstein MT, Tucci V, Isenberg HD, Singer C: Central catheter infections: single- versus triple-lumen catheters. Influence of guide wires on infection rates when used for replacement of catheters. Am J Med 1988;84:667–672.

153 Clark-Christoff N, Watters VA, Sparks W, Snyder P, Grant JP: Use of triple-lumen subclavian catheters for administration of total parenteral nutrition. JPEN J Parenter Enteral Nutr 1992;16:403–407.

154 Michelson AD, Bovill E, Monagle P, Andrew M: Antithrombotic therapy in children. Chest 1998;114(suppl):748S–769S.

155 Randolph AG, Cook DJ, Gonzales CA, Andrew M: Benefit of heparin in central venous and pulmonary artery catheters: a meta-analysis of randomized controlled trials. Chest 1998;113:165–171.

156 Smith S, Dawson S, Hennessey R, Andrew M: Maintenance of the patency of indwelling central venous catheters: is heparin necessary? Am J Pediatr Hematol Oncol 1991;13:141–143.

157 de Neef M, Heijboer H, van Woensel JB, de Haan RJ: The efficacy of heparinization in prolonging patency of arterial and central venous catheters in children: a randomized double-blind trial. Pediatr Hematol Oncol 2002;19:553–560.

158 Kamala F, Boo NY, Cheah FC, Birinder K: Randomized controlled trial of heparin for prevention of blockage of peripherally inserted central catheters in neonates. Acta Paediatr 2002; 91:1350–1356.

159 Maki DG, Ringer M, Alvarado CJ: Prospective randomised trial of povidone-iodine, alcohol, and chlorhexidine for prevention of infection associated with central venous and arterial catheters. Lancet 1991;338:339–343.

160 Hoffmann KK, Weber DJ, Samsa GP, Rutala WA: Transparent polyurethane film as an intravenous catheter dressing. A meta-analysis of the infection risks. JAMA 1992;267:2072–2076.

161 Taylor D, Myers ST, Monarch K, Leon C, Hall J, Sibley Y: Use of occlusive dressings on central venous catheter sites in hospitalized children. J Pediatr Nurs 1996;11:169–174.

162 Mascarenhas MR, Zemel B, Stallings VA: Nutritional assessment in pediatrics. Nutrition 1998;14:105–115.

163 Williamson RC: Intestinal adaptation (first of two parts). Structural, functional and cytokinetic changes. N Engl J Med 1978;298:1393–1402.

164 Levine GM, Deren JJ, Steiger E, Zinno R: Role of oral intake in maintenance of gut mass and disaccharide activity. Gastroenterology 1974;67:975–982.

165 Greene HL, McCabe DR, Merenstein GB: Protracted diarrhea and malnutrition in infancy: changes in intestinal morphology and disaccharidase activities during treatment with total intravenous nutrition or oral elemental diets. J Pediatr 1975;87:695–704.

166 Johnson LR, Copeland EM, Dudrick SJ, Lichtenberger LM, Castro GA: Structural and hormonal alterations in the gastrointestinal tract of parenterally fed rats. Gastroenterology 1975;68:1177–1183.

167 Feldman EJ, Dowling RH, McNaughton J, Peters TJ: Effects of oral versus intravenous nutrition on intestinal adaptation after small bowel resection in the dog. Gastroenterology 1976;70:712–719.

168 Andorsky DJ, Lund DP, Lillehei CW, Jaksic T, Dicanzio J, Richardson DS, et al: Nutritional and other postoperative management of neonates with short bowel syndrome correlates with clinical outcomes. J Pediatr 2001;139:27–33.

169 Strudwick S: Gastro-oesophageal reflux and feeding: the speech and language therapist's perspective. Int J Pediatr Otorhinolaryngol 2003;67(suppl 1):S101–S102.

170 Puntis JW, Wilkins KM, Ball PA, Rushton DI, Booth IW: Hazards of parenteral treatment: do particles count? Arch Dis Child 1992;67:1475–1477.

171 Vargas JH, Ament ME, Berquist WE: Long-term home parenteral nutrition in pediatrics: ten years of experience in 102 patients. J Pediatr Gastroenterol Nutr 1987;6:24–32.

172 Colomb V, Talbotec C, Goulet O, et al: Outcome in children on long term-(home)-parenteral nutrition: a 20 year-experience. Clin Nutr 2003;22:73–74.

173 Liptak GS: Home care for children who have chronic conditions. Pediatr Rev 1997;18:271–273.

174 Stokes MA, Almond DJ, Pettit SH, Mughal MM, Turner M, Shaffer JL, et al: Home parenteral nutrition: a review of 100 patient years of treatment in 76 consecutive cases. Br J Surg
1988;75:481–483.

175 Ricour C, Gorski AM, Goulet O: Home parenteral nutrition in children: 8 years of experience
with 112 patients. Clin Nutr 1990;9:65–71.

176 Bisset WM, Stapleford P, Long S, Chamberlain A, Sokel B, Milla PJ: Home parenteral nutrition in chronic intestinal failure. Arch Dis Child 1992;67:109–114.

177 Puntis JW: Home parenteral nutrition. Arch Dis Child 1995;72:186–190.

178 Phillips LD: Patient education. Understanding the process to maximize time and outcomes.
J Intraven Nurs 1999;22:19–35.

179 Meadows N: Home parenteral nutrition in children. Bailleres Clin Pediatr 1997;5:189–199.

180 Stokes DC, Rao BN, Mirro J Jr, Mackert PW, Austin B, Colten M, et al: Early detection and
simplified management of obstructed Hickman and Broviac catheters. J Pediatr Surg
1989;24:257–262.

181 Holcombe BJ, Forloines-Lynn S, Garmhausen LW: Restoring patency of long-term central
venous access devices. J Intraven Nurs 1992;15:36–41.

182 Glynn MF, Langer B, Jeejeebhoy KN: Therapy for thrombotic occlusion of long-term intravenous alimentation catheters. JPEN J Parenter Enteral Nutr 1980;4:387–390.

183 Hurtubise MR, Bottino JC, Lawson M, McCredie KB: Restoring patency of occluded central
venous catheters. Arch Surg 1980;115:212–213.

184 Shulman RJ, Reed T, Pitre D, Laine L: Use of hydrochloric acid to clear obstructed central
venous catheters. JPEN J Parenter Enteral Nutr 1988;12:509–510.

185 Duffy LF, Kerzner B, Gebus V, Dice J: Treatment of central venous catheter occlusions with
hydrochloric acid. J Pediatr 1989;114:1002–1004.

186 Wachs T: Urokinase administration in pediatric patients with occluded central venous catheters. J Intraven Nurs 1990;13:100–102.

187 Werlin SL, Lausten T, Jessen S, Toy L, Norton A, Dallman L, et al: Treatment of central venous
catheter occlusions with ethanol and hydrochloric acid. JPEN J Parenter Enteral Nutr
1995;19:416–418.

188 Harris JL, Maguire D: Developing a protocol to prevent and treat pediatric central venous
catheter occlusions. J Intraven Nurs 1999;22:194–198.

189 Choi M, Massicotte MP, Marzinotto V, Chan AK, Holmes JL, Andrew M: The use of alteplase
to restore patency of central venous lines in pediatric patients: a cohort study. J Pediatr 2001;
139:152–156.

190 Crain MR, Horton MG, Mewissen MW: Fibrin sheaths complicating central venous catheters. AJR Am J Roentgenol 1998;171:341–346.

191 Smith VC, Hallett JW Jr: Subclavian vein thrombosis during prolonged catheterization for
parenteral nutrition: early management and long-term follow-up. South Med J 1983;76:603–
606.

192 Mughal MM: Complications of intravenous feeding catheters. Br J Surg 1989;76:15–21.

193 Grant J: Recognition, prevention, and treatment of home total parenteral nutrition central
venous access complications. JPEN J Parenter Enteral Nutr 2002;26(suppl):S21–S28.

194 Bern MM, Lokich JJ, Wallach SR, Bothe A Jr, Benotti PN, Arkin CF, et al: Very low doses of warfarin can prevent thrombosis in central venous catheters. A randomized prospective trial. Ann Intern Med 1990;112:423–428.

195 Veerabagu MP, Tuttle-Newhall J, Maliakkal R, Champagne C, Mascioli EA: Warfarin and reduced central venous thrombosis in home total parenteral nutrition patients. Nutrition 1995;11:142–144.

196 Monreal M, Alastrue A, Rull M, Mira X, Muxart J, Rosell R, et al: Upper extremity deep venous thrombosis in cancer patients with venous access devices – prophylaxis with a low molecular weight heparin (Fragmin). Thromb Haemost 1996;75:251–253.

197 Barnett MI, Cosslett AG, Duffield JR, Evans DA, Hall SB, Williams DR: Parenteral nutrition. Pharmaceutical problems of compatibility and stability. Drug Saf 1990;5(suppl 1):101–106.

198 Pluhator-Murton MM, Fedorak RN, Audette RJ, Marriage BJ, Yatscoff RW: Extent of trace-element contamination from simulated compounding of total parenteral nutrient solutions. Am J Health Syst Pharm 1996;53:2299–2303.

199 Pluhator-Murton MM, Fedorak RN, Audette RJ, Marriage BJ, Yatscoff RW, Gramlich LM: Trace element contamination of total parenteral nutrition. 1. Contribution of component solutions. JPEN J Parenter Enteral Nutr 1999;23:222–227.

200 Pluhator-Murton MM, Fedorak RN, Audette RJ, Marriage BJ, Yatscoff RW, Gramlich LM: Trace element contamination of total parenteral nutrition. 2. Effect of storage duration and temperature. JPEN J Parenter Enteral Nutr 1999;23:228–232.

201 Murphy S, Craig DQ, Murphy A: An investigation into the physical stability of a neonatal parenteral nutrition formulation. Acta Paediatr 1996;85:1483–1486.

202 Barnett MI, Cosslett AG, Minton A: The interaction of heparin, calcium and lipid emulsions in simulated Y-site delivery of total parenteral nutrition (TPN) admixtures. Clin Nutr 1996; 15:49.

203 Durand MC, Barnett MI: Heparin in parenteral feeding: effect of heparin and low molecular weight heparin on lipid emulsions and all-in-one admixtures. Br J Intens Care 1992;2: 10–12.

204 Lumpkin MM: Safety alert: hazards of precipitation associated with parenteral nutrition. Am J Hosp Pharm 1994;51:1427–1428.

205 Dellert SF, Farrell MK, Specker BL, Heubi JE: Bone mineral content in children with short bowel syndrome after discontinuation of parental nutrition. J Pediatr 1998;132:516–519.

206 Leonberg BL, Chuang E, Eicher P, Tershakovec AM, Leonard L, Stallings VA: Long-term growth and development in children after home parental nutrition. J Pediatr 1998;132:461–466.

207 Nousia-Arvanitakis S, Angelopoulou-Sakadami N, Metroliou K: Complications associated with total parenteral nutrition in infants with short bowel syndrome. Hepatogastroenterology 1992;39:169–172.

208 Advenier E, Landry C, Colomb V, Cognon C, Pradeau D, Florent M, et al: Aluminum contamination of parenteral nutrition and aluminum loading in children on long-term parenteral nutrition. J Pediatr Gastroenterol Nutr 2003;36:448–453.

209 Fouin-Fortunet H, Le Quernec L, Erlinger S, Lerebours E, Colin R: Hepatic alterations during total parenteral nutrition in patients with inflammatory bowel disease: a possible consequence of lithocholate toxicity. Gastroenterology 1982;82:932–937.

210 Quigley EM, Marsh MN, Shaffer JL, Markin RS: Hepatobiliary complications of total parenteral nutrition. Gastroenterology 1993;104:286–301.

211 Kwan V, George J: Liver disease due to parenteral and enteral nutrition. Clin Liver Dis 2004;8(4):893–913, ix–x.

212 Forbes A: Parenteral nutrition: new advances and observations. Curr Opin Gastroenterol 2004;20:114–118.

Subject Index